GIRLY RECIPES

Very Easy!

Ruby Fry

Contents

Chapter One

toasted nuts and smoked gouda salad with turkey and cranberries

Serves 4 people 20-minute prep time

Our Thanksgiving tradition has always been to have open-faced turkey sandwiches with mashed potatoes, crumbs of stuffing, hot gravy, and a glob of cranberry sauce the day after Thanksgiving. As much as I enjoy the sparkle and shine of that obscenely wonderful dish, I'm also ready to eat a little lighter the day after Thanksgiving. This salad dish comes in handy in that situation. With roasted turkey and dried cranberries, it's reminiscent of Thanksgiving, but with the addition of smoked Gouda and apple, it's elevated. After filling yourself with stuffing, serve it all on a bed of fresh spinach with a little vinaigrette to help you get back on track.

DRESSING

2 teaspoons vegetable or canola oil

apple cider vinegar, 2 tablespoons

1 tablespoon shallot, finely chopped

1 tablespoon lemon juice, freshly squeezed

1 teaspoon maple sugar

1 teaspoon of salt

1/8 teaspoon black pepper, freshly ground

SALAD

8 cups spinach (baby)

12 cup roasted turkey, diced

1 cored and chopped large Red Delicious apple (unpeeled)

34 cup 12-inch smoked Gouda cheese cubes

12 cup cranberries, dried

12 cup toasted chopped walnuts (see Tips)

To make the dressing, mix together the dressing ingredients in a small bowl.

To make the salad, combine all of the salad ingredients in a large mixing bowl.

Toss the salad with the dressing. Serve right away.

ADAPTABLE WITHOUT GLUTEN Make sure to use a gluten-free maple syrup. Check to see if your roasted turkey has any gluten.

ADAPTABLE DAIRY-FREE Remove the cheese.

TIP Preheat the oven to 350°F for toasting the walnuts. On a baking sheet, spread the walnuts out. 3 to 5 minutes in the oven, just until they are gently browned and fragrant. If you leave them in the oven for too long, they will go from toasted to burnt in a matter of minutes or seconds.

Instead of turkey, use roasted chicken and dried currants instead of cranberries.

Instead of roasted walnuts, use sugared walnuts: Place the walnuts in a small skillet. 14 cup granulated white sugar, heated over medium heat Stir constantly until the sugar has melted and the walnuts have been coated. Remove the nuts from the heat and spread them out to cool on a baking sheet. Break up the nuts and toss them into the salad.

Chapter Two

romaine lettuce grilled with blue cheese, tomato, and bacon

Serves 4 people Time to Prepare: 25 minutes 5 minutes to prepare

My obsession with all things bacon is almost as strong as my passion for blue cheese. I enjoy breaking off bits and eating it on its own, pairing it with fresh figs and honey for an appetiser, and tossing it into risotto or nibbling it with roast meat. But it's in salads that I really enjoy blue cheese. This salad takes the best of both worlds and blends bacon and blue cheese together.

DRESSING

14 cup crumbled blue cheese

1 tablespoon mayonnaise

2 tbsp lemon juice, freshly squeezed

To taste, season with salt and freshly ground black pepper.

GREENS

four romaine hearts (see Tips)

2 tbsp olive oil extra-virgin

freshly ground black pepper and salt

TOPPINGS

6 slices bacon, cooked till crisp and crumbled (see Tips)

1 pint halved cherry or pear tomatoes (about 2 cups)

blue cheese crumbles (optional)

To make the dressing, combine the blue cheese, mayonnaise, lemon juice, salt, and pepper in a medium mixing bowl, pressing the blue cheese crumbles into the mayonnaise. Refrigerate the dressing in the bowl covered in plastic wrap while you finish the remainder of the salad.

Preheat your grill to medium. Grates should be oiled.

To make the greens, spray olive oil over the romaine hearts and season with salt and pepper. Place the romaine on the grill and cook for 3 to 4 minutes, or until it is slightly browned and wilted on all sides. Place each romaine heart on a serving tray after removing it from the grill.

Dressing, bacon, tomatoes, and blue cheese crumbles go on top of each romaine heart.

ADAPTABLE WITHOUT GLUTEN Replace the blue cheese with feta or goat cheese, and use gluten-free mayonnaise and bacon.

TIPS The centre leaves of romaine lettuce are known as romaine hearts. In the produce department of your supermarket, look for them packaged.

Cook your bacon in the oven for simple cleanup. Preheat the oven to 400 degrees Fahrenheit. Place a rack on top of a big, rimmed baking sheet lined with foil. Using nonstick spray, coat the rack. On the rack, arrange the bacon strips. Bake for 15 to 20 minutes, or until crisp. The length of time depends on how thick your bacon is.

If you don't like blue cheese, substitute feta or goat cheese instead.

If you don't want to grill the romaine, chop it up and serve with the same toppings as before.

Chapter Three

Salad of diced chicken and couscous with a basil dressing

Serves 4 people 35-minute prep time

Chopped salads have been around for a long time, usually in the form of an Italian chopped or a chopped Cobb. I personally enjoy salads that are "chopped." Because everything is diced tiny, there's a considerable probability that all of the salad ingredients will fit into a single forkful. This implies that each bite contains all of the flavours of the entire salad. I have a great to-go salad that I get whenever I can at one of my favourite markets (Trader Joe's). I'm infatuated with the crunch and sweetness of it all, and if it's cut finely enough, each bite contains the entire salad. Here's how I make that favourite salad at home.

DRESSING

1 pound mayonnaise

2 tablespoons fresh basil, finely chopped

1 tablespoon pesto sauce (prepared)

1 teaspoon of water

2 tablespoons lemon juice, freshly squeezed

1 tblsp. honey

1 teaspoon of salt

1/8 teaspoon black pepper, freshly ground

SALAD

4 cups romaine lettuce, finely chopped

2 cups roasted chicken, coarsely chopped

2 cups kernels of corn (see Tips)

2 cups red cabbage, finely chopped

1 cup dried Israeli couscous, cooked and cooled according to package recommendations (see Tips)

1 medium red bell pepper, seeded and coarsely chopped (ribs removed).

12 cup Parmesan cheese, freshly grated

12 cup currants, dry

12 cup pecans, finely chopped

To make the dressing, mix together the dressing ingredients in a small bowl. If the dressing is too thick, whisk add a teaspoon of water at a time until you reach the desired consistency. It should be rich and creamy, yet pourable as well.

To make the salad, combine all of the salad ingredients in a large mixing bowl.

Toss in the dressing to coat. Serve the salad in four separate bowls.

TIP This salad is fantastic with fresh corn. Simply chop the corn kernels off the cob and toss them into the salad raw. 2 cups corn kernels should be enough from two large cobs.

Israeli couscous (also known as pearl couscous) is twice the size of conventional couscous and is roasted rather than dried. This gives it a nutty flavour and a chewy bite, making it more suitable for adding into salads where it may compete with the other salad ingredients. You can usually find Israeli couscous anywhere regular couscous is sold.

If you like, place the salad dressing on the side so that each person can garnish their own salad.

Use diced turkey instead of chicken, wild rice instead of couscous, and dried cranberries instead of currants to make a salad for the day after Thanksgiving.

Chapter Four

Arugula, white wine, and whole grain mustard gruyère grilled cheese

Approximately 1 sandwich 15-minute prep time Time to cook: 8 minutes

Grilled cheese is the epitome of comfort food. Anyone can feel happy with all that melting cheese. Even a simple toasted cheese and buttered bread sandwich can make one's heart skip a beat. I've made an adult version for you. This sandwich also includes a smidgeon of cream cheese, a splash of white wine, and peppery arugula. It should provide you with plenty of relief.

1 tablespoon room temperature salted butter

2 bread slices (see Tips)

12 tsp. white wine (see Tips)

12 tablespoon mustard (whole grain)

4 thin Gruyère or Swiss cheese slices, divided

arugula, 13 cup

2 thin tomato slices

1 tablespoon cream cheese, softened

12 tbsp butter, spread on each slice of bread Place the bread slices on a chopping board butter side down. One slice should be brushed with white wine and then mustard. Cover the entire piece of bread with two slices of Gruyère, breaking it apart as needed. On top of the Gruyère, layer the arugula and tomato. Place the remaining Gruyère slices on top of the tomato. Spread cream cheese on the second slice of bread and set it on top of the tomato, cream cheese side down.

Spray a skillet with nonstick spray and heat to medium. Cover the sandwich in the skillet with the lid. Reduce the heat to a low setting. Cook for 3 to 4 minutes, then remove the lid and peek underneath the sandwich with a spatula. Flip the sandwich over when the bottom has turned golden brown. Cover the skillet and cook for another 3 to 4 minutes, or until the opposite side is golden as well. Remove the pan from the heat and set the sandwich in the hot pan for 2 minutes. Place the sandwich on a cutting board and cut it in half before serving.

TIPS For this grilled cheese sandwich, I use thin-sliced French or sourdough bread.

If you don't want to use alcohol in the sandwich, leave it out.

In this sandwich, use your favourite types of cheese. It's delicious with provolone, Jack, or cheddar cheese.

Prosciutto, bacon, and Dijon mustard are also excellent grilled cheese toppings.

Chapter Five

jerked pork sandwiches with root beer

Approximately 10 sandwiches Time to Prepare: 25 minutes 11 hours and 30 minutes to cook

There was one thing I craved more than anything else while I was pregnant with my son: root beer. I looked everywhere for the best root beer in the land. I tried both artisan and generic varieties. Mug was at the centre of it all. The one that appeared to satiate my hunger the best was mug root beer. I still crave it now that I'm not pregnant, and it also works well as a cooking marinade for pulled pork. This meal will feed a large group or a hungry family for several days.

1 bone-in pork shoulder butt roast, 5 to 6 pounds

1 ounce dried onion soup mix envelope

freshly ground black pepper and salt

1 root beer 12-ounce can (I prefer Mug brand)

2 cups barbecue sauce (distributed)

10 hamburger buns, normal size, your choice

Remove any excess fat from the pork roast. It's fine to leave some on there as long as the large, obvious slabs are removed. Sprinkle the onion soup mix over the roast and place it on a work surface. Rub the mixture into the meat with clean hands, reaching below to coat both sides. Season with salt and pepper to taste. In your slow cooker, place the seasoned roast.

Whisk together the root beer and 12 cup barbecue sauce in a medium mixing basin. In the slow cooker, pour over the roast.

Cook for 10 to 11 hours on low heat, or until the internal temperature reaches 190°F and the meat begins to peel away from the bone. Transfer the roast to a chopping board and set aside to cool. All but about 34 cup of the slow cooker fluids should be poured out and discarded. Shred the pork with two forks, cutting around and eliminating any fatty bits. Return all of the pulled pork to the slow cooker, along with any remaining juices. Add the remaining 112 cup barbecue sauce to the pan. Replace the cover and stir to blend. Cook for 15 to 20 minutes over high heat, or until the pork and fluids are heated and bubbling. Preheat the oven to 200°F in the meantime. Place the cut side up on a baking sheet after splitting the buns. Warm the dish in the oven until ready to serve.

Place the pulled pork on the warmed buns and serve right away.

TIPS If you don't want to cook such a huge roast, you may prepare a smaller roast using the same components. Reduce the cooking time by a few minutes and use less barbecue sauce before serving.

I don't advocate trying to shorten the recipe by cooking it on high heat for tender pulled pork. It's best to go slow and steady.

Cola can be substituted for root beer.

To make a deli-style sandwich, pile coleslaw on top of the pulled pork.

Lobster rolls with a hint of lemon

Preparation time: 10 minutes yields 2 lobster rolls

The lobster roll is a New England specialty that can be prepared in a variety of ways. What right does a Californian have to teach the rest of the world how to cook a lobster roll? Almost certainly none. But every summer, I spend a few weeks in Massachusetts, where lobsters are frequently boiled and ripped apart into lobster rolls in my kitchen. Mine is fairly straightforward. To complement the amazing lobster flavour, a few flavours should be added. The greatest lobster rolls are served with potato chips and a cold beer.

2 cups cooked lobster meat, diced

2 tblsp. mayonnaise

a sprinkling of salt

2 freshly ground black peppercorns

1 teaspoon lemon juice, freshly squeezed

12 teaspoon lemon zest, grated

2 toasted hot dog rolls (see Tips)

Combine the lobster, mayonnaise, salt, pepper, lemon juice, and zest in a medium mixing bowl.

Serve the lobster filling immediately between the two hot dog buns.

TIPS I like to toast the buns by brushing them with melted butter and frying them butter side down in a large, hot skillet.

If you live in New England, take advantage of the delicious New England style hot dog buns that are readily available. Use your preferred type of hot dog bun for the rest of the world.

To give your sandwich some crunch, add chopped celery and green onions.

Hot dogs with avocado and creamy chipotle sauce

Prep Time: 15 minutes Cook Time: 10 minutes Yield: 8 hot dogs

I have the ideal hot dog for avocado fans. Some may find the thought of putting avocado on a hot dog weird. But if you're a fan of this velvety green fruit, you'll have to believe me. My own husband used to be a sceptic, but now he's unhappy if I just produce regular dogs. These hot dogs have a mild chipotle sauce, tomato, avocado, and Cojita, a salty crumbled Mexican cheese.

SAUCE WITH CHIPOTLES

a quarter-cup of mayonnaise

2 teaspoons adobo chipotle sauce (see Tips)

HOT DOGS

8 hot dogs of decent quality (I prefer Hebrew National or Nathan's)

8 buns for hot dogs

4 tablespoons salted butter (12 stick) at room temperature

1 cup tomato, chopped

2 pitted, peeled, and chopped avocados

12 cup Cojita cheese, crumbled (see Tips)

Preheat your grill to medium.

To make the chipotle sauce, whisk together the mayonnaise and chipotle sauce in a medium mixing basin. Cover the bowl with plastic wrap and chill until ready to assemble the hot dogs.

Grill the hot dogs for 5 to 7 minutes, turning frequently, until they have grill marks on all sides. Meanwhile, butter each bun with 12 tablespoons of butter. Grill the buns with the butter side down on the cooler sides of the grill. When the buns are gently browned, about 1 to 2 minutes, remove them from the grill.

To make the sandwiches, lay a hot dog in each toasted bread and top with 112 tablespoons chipotle sauce. Serve the dogs immediately with the tomato, avocados, and cheese.

TIPS Chipotle sauce is the adobo sauce contained in chipotle chiles in a can. It can be found in your market's Latin-American items area. If you want it really hot, add some chopped chipotles! Divide the remaining chipotle peppers and sauce among a few zip baggies and store in the freezer for up to 6 months.

If you don't have a grill, boil or fry the hot dogs and toast the buns in the oven.

Cojita cheese is a spherical Latin-American cheese that is frequently available beside cream cheese in the supermarket. Feta or goat cheese can also be used.

Toss your hot dogs with chopped fresh cilantro.

Monte Cristo sandwiches with prosciutto and brie

Prep Time: 25 minutes Cook Time: 5 minutes Yield: 4 sandwiches

I was recently sitting in a lunchtime restaurant, perusing my menu options. I was initially interested when I saw a Monte Cristo sandwich. It had a catchy name, was fried in an egg batter, and was served with jam for dipping. I had never seen anything like it before and decided to order it for lunch. I fell in love with that sandwich and haven't been able to get it out of my mind. It's no surprise that I included a rendition of it in this collection.

8 34-inch challah slices (about three-quarters of a 1-pound loaf) (see Tips)

2 tablespoons mustard (whole grain)

8 ounces sliced Brie

4 prosciutto slices or thinly sliced ham

1 percent milk, 34 cup

three huge eggs

2 tblsp salted butter (divided)

14 cup raspberry jam (seedless)

On a cutting board, arrange four slices of bread. 12 tbsp mustard, spread on each slice Top each slice of bread with cheese and prosciutto, then a second slice of bread.

Whisk together the milk and eggs in a medium mixing basin.

1 tablespoon butter, melted in a large skillet over medium heat Coat both sides of one of the sandwiches with the egg batter. In a heated skillet, place the sandwich. Continue with the second sandwich. Cook the sandwiches for 3 to 4 minutes, or until golden brown on the underside. Cook for an additional 2 to 3 minutes on the other side, or until golden brown on both sides. Place the sandwiches on a serving plate. Replace the butter, sandwiches, and egg batter as needed. Warm raspberry jam is served alongside.

TIP Good bread is an important component of this sandwich's success. Don't make the mistake of using standard sandwich bread. Challah, brioche, or any other herb-free, sliceable bread would suffice.

Prosciutto can be replaced with thinly sliced turkey or ham.

If you like, you can replace the Brie with Havarti cheese. Another fantastic melting cheese that goes well in this sandwich is Havarti.

Turkey sliders with bacon, avocado, and barbecue sauce cooked from scratch

Prep Time: 40 minutes Cook Time: 35 minutes Yield: 12 sliders

If you're unfamiliar with the term "slider," it's basically a cute, little burger. Because three sliders are around the same size as a larger burger, eating multiples is okay. Ground turkey and sweet Italian sausage are combined to make these sliders. Only one is possible with a smidgeon of homemade barbeque sauce, a strip of crispy bacon, and sliced avocado on top.

BURGERS

34 pound turkey ground

12 pound Italian sweet sausage

a third of a cup of bread crumbs

milk, 3 tablespoons

1 big, lightly beaten egg

2 teaspoons garlic, minced

freshly ground black pepper and salt

BUNS AND TOPPINGS

12 2 inch sharp cheddar cheese slices

12 mini dinner rolls or 12 slider buns

3 bacon slices, quartered and fried till crisp (see Tips)

1 large avocado, peeled, pitted, and thinly sliced

SAUCE FOR BARBECUE

1 ketchup cup

14 cup of apple cider vinegar

molasses (1 tablespoon)

1 teaspoon of honey

1 tablespoon mustard (Dijon)

1 teaspoon of water

12 teaspoon sauce de Worcester

12 teaspoon sodium chloride

12 teaspoon black pepper, freshly ground

Preheat the oven to 400 degrees Fahrenheit. Using nonstick spray, coat a large, rimmed baking sheet.

To make the burgers, combine all of the ingredients in a medium mixing bowl. Gently mix the ingredients together with a fork until they are fully blended. Form the meat into twelve 3- to 4-inch patties on the prepared baking sheet, using approximately 13 cup each burger. Bake for 30 to 35 minutes, or until the burgers are golden brown and cooked through.

To make the barbecue sauce, whisk together all of the sauce ingredients in a medium saucepan over medium-high heat until well mixed. Bring to a boil, then reduce to a low heat and continue to cook for 10 minutes. Keep heated until ready to serve with the sliders.

To make the sliders, top each burger with a slice of cheese and cook for an additional 1 to 2 minutes in the oven, just until the cheese has melted. Distribute the sauce evenly among the ten buns. Add a slider, a slice of bacon, and one or two slices of avocado to the top. Serve right away.

TIP While the burgers are baking, fry the bacon in a medium skillet over medium heat for 6 to 8 minutes, or until crisp. Drain the bacon on a dish lined with paper towels.

TIP: Make the barbecue sauce up to 2 days ahead of time. Keep it chilled and covered. Form the burger patties and set them on the baking sheet the day before you plan to serve them. Cover the patties with plastic wrap and keep them refrigerated until ready to bake.

QUICK AND EASY TIP: Instead of making your own barbecue sauce, buy some.

Instead of baking the sliders, grill them. Grill them for 3 to 4 minutes per side over medium heat, or until cooked through.

Other options for slider toppings include grilled onions, tomatoes, peperoncini, and other cheeses.

wraps with buffalo chicken

Prep Time: 25 minutes Cook Time: 7 minutes Yield: 4 wraps

Buffalo wings remind me of my college days. Near campus, there was a dive-restaurant dedicated to serving up the most delectable spicy wings, complete with blue cheese dressing and celery sticks. College reminds me of how many wings I ate during those days, which undoubtedly contributed to my Freshman Fifteen. That wing consumption makes me want I still had access to those wings, and this Buffalo Chicken Wraps recipe is a sandwich version of that wish.

DRESSING WITH BLUE CHEESE

13 cup crumbled blue cheese

1 pound mayonnaise

2 tbsp lemon juice, freshly squeezed

To taste, season with salt and freshly ground black pepper.

THE FINAL INGREDIENTS

1 cup of liquid

12 cup rice, white

1 pound chopped into 1-inch chunks chicken tenders

cayenne pepper sauce (13 cup) (see Tips)

4 big warmed wheat tortillas or wraps

12 cup iceberg lettuce, chopped

1 cup celery, chopped

1 cup tomato, finely chopped

Optional extra cayenne pepper sauce

To make the dressing, combine the blue cheese, mayonnaise, lemon juice, and a pinch of salt and pepper in a medium mixing bowl. Set aside or refrigerate the dressing until you're ready to assemble your wraps.

In a small saucepan over high heat, bring the water to a boil for the following ingredients. Toss in the rice. Cook, covered, over medium heat until the rice is cooked and has absorbed all of the liquid, about 20 minutes.

Heat a medium skillet over medium heat with nonstick spray. 3 to 4 minutes per side, add the chicken to the heated skillet and cook until lightly browned on all sides and no longer pink on the interior. Remove the chicken from the pan and combine it with the cayenne pepper sauce in a medium mixing bowl.

Wrap the tortillas in damp paper towels and microwave for 40 seconds to assemble the wraps. Place the tortillas on a flat work surface and divide the chicken tenders amongst them. Evenly distribute the rice, lettuce, celery, and tomato between the tortillas. Each wrap should have 112 tablespoons of dressing. If desired, drizzle with extra hot sauce.

Fold the bottom fourth of the wrap over the bottom fourth of the tortilla. Fold the left and right sides over the filling and hold them together to keep them together (see Tips).

TIPS I recommend Frank's brand cayenne pepper sauce for the cayenne pepper sauce, but you can also use a sauce made specifically for Buffalo wings.

This wrap benefits from the crunchiness of iceberg lettuce, but you may use any chopped lettuce you choose.

Take a piece of foil and wrap it around the bottom half of each wrap to help hold it together as you wrap each sandwich. This also makes eating easier because the filling won't have to fight its way out of the bottom of the tortillas.

If you don't like blue cheese, use Ranch dressing instead and top your wrap with shredded cheddar cheese.

Avocado lovers may want to include some freshly sliced avocado.

Sandwiches with peppers and caramelised onions made in the slow cooker

Prep Time: 45 minutes Cook Time: 12 hours Makes: 8 big sandwiches

When I was approximately 12 years old, I learnt how to roast beef. When I got home from school, Mom would lightly season the roast and put it in the refrigerator for me to put in the oven. When mother got home from work, she'd make mashed potatoes, gravy, and steamed peas or corn, and we'd have a filling dinner for my older, adolescent brother. With the leftovers, we nearly always made French Dip Sandwiches, getting at least two dinners out of the same roast. This recipe simplifies the roasting of meat. The beef comes out as soft as can be after being cooked in the slow cooker.

BEEF

4 pound boneless beef roast with extra fat removed

1 tablespoon garlic, minced (2 large cloves)

1 tablespoon fresh rosemary, minced (or 1 teaspoon dried)

1 tablespoon fresh thyme, minced (or 1 teaspoon dried)

1 teaspoon salt (kosher)

12 teaspoon black pepper, freshly ground

2 low-sodium beef broth 14.5-ounce cans

1 tbsp. Worcestershire

10 peppercorns, whole

1 bay leaf

12 medium onion, chopped into bits

ONIONS CARAMELIZED

2 tablespoons extra virgin olive oil

2 big finely sliced onions

1 teaspoon salt (kosher)

PEPPERS

1 large red bell pepper, seeded and chopped into thin strips (ribs removed).

1 large green bell pepper, seeded and chopped into thin strips (ribs removed).

THE FINAL INGREDIENTS

8 6-inch French sandwich rolls with a crust

4 tablespoons salted butter, softened (12 stick)

8 provolone cheese slices

In your slow cooker, place the roast. Combine the garlic, rosemary, thyme, salt, and pepper in a small bowl. Rub the spice mixture into the roast with clean fingertips. Around the sides of the roast, pour the beef broth. If the roast Isn't completely buried in the broth, fill the slow cooker with just enough water to cover it. Combine the Worcestershire sauce, peppercorns, and bay leaf in a mixing bowl. On top of the roast, place the onion. Cover and cook on low for 11 to 12 hours, or until the meat flakes apart easily with a fork.

Prepare the caramelised onions and peppers in the last hour of cooking. Heat the olive oil in a large skillet over medium heat. Cook, turning frequently, until the onions are golden brown, about 30 minutes, decreasing heat as needed if the onions are burning or browning too quickly. If the pan becomes too dry, add 1 tablespoon of water. The onions will turn a rich golden brown colour and have a delicious flavour. Wipe clean the pan and transfer the onions to a serving bowl. Add the bell peppers to the pan and cook over medium heat. Cook, stirring frequently, for about 7 minutes, or until the peppers have softened. Place the peppers in a separate serving bowl.

Transfer the meat to a chopping board from the slow cooker. Cut the meat against the grain into slices or shred it with a fork. Using a fine sieve, strain the broth from the slow cooker into a bowl. Allow the broth to cool to room temperature to allow the fat to separate.

Preheat the broiler in the oven. Dividing the rolls 12 tablespoon butter should be spread on the cut side of the rolls. Place the rolls on a rimmed baking sheet open-faced. 2 to 3 minutes under the broiler, or until golden brown. Take the rolls out of the oven and top with meat, caramelised onions, peppers, and a slice of cheese. Return the sandwiches to the oven and broil for 1 to 2 minutes more, or until the cheese has melted. Skim any accumulated fat from the surface of the broth with a spoon. Fill cups halfway with broth. Serve toasted sandwiches with dipping bowls of broth.

TIPS While the caramelised onions and peppers are tasty complements to the sandwich, they are not required. Serve meat and cheese sandwiches for a more straightforward option.

To serve these at noon (excellent for athletic events!), start them late at night and finish them by lunchtime the next day.

Instead of serving these in dinner rolls, turn them into French Dip Sliders.

For those who like things spicy, keep a bottle of hot sauce nearby.

Tacos with flank steak and avocado-chimichurri sauce

Makes 12 tacos Prep Time: 25 minutes Plus time to marinate Cook Time: 10 minutes

Millie, a Peruvian acquaintance, and her husband David routinely hold dinner parties in their lawn in California, where they serve a variety of South American dishes. They know how to cook and appreciate delicious cuisine. Millie taught me how to make empanadas, and her husband gave me some pointers on how to slow-grill the most wonderfully seasoned meats I've ever had. In his wood-fired oven, David roasts an unlimited variety of veggies and meats. His grilled flank steak with chimichurri sauce is my personal favourite. These tacos were inspired by that.

STEAK

1 tablespoon extra virgin olive oil

2 medium limes, grated zest and juice

3 minced medium garlic cloves

honey, 2 teaspoons

2 tablespoons cumin powder

12 teaspoon sodium chloride

12 teaspoon black pepper, freshly ground

2 pound flank steak or skirt steak, fat removed and discarded

SAUCE DE CHIMICHURRI

1 cup cilantro, chopped

14 cup vinegar (red wine)

2 tablespoons extra virgin olive oil

2 minced medium garlic cloves

1 tblsp. honey

12 teaspoon cumin powder

12 teaspoon red pepper, crushed

a quarter teaspoon of salt

12 large pitted and peeled avocados

TO BE SERVED

12 reheated or fried corn or taco-size flour tortillas (see Tips)

3 cups iceberg lettuce, chopped

12 cup Monterey Jack cheese, shredded

12 quarts salsa

To marinate the steak, put the olive oil, lime zest, lime juice, garlic, honey, cumin, salt, and pepper in a big zip baggie or glass dish. Toss in the steak and turn it a couple times to coat it with the marinade. While you're making the sauce, let the steak sit at room temperature for 30 minutes.

To make the sauce, put the cilantro, vinegar, oil, garlic, honey, cumin, crushed red pepper, and sea salt in a blender or small food processor. Process the ingredients for 1 minute, or until well blended. Process until the sauce is smooth, adding the avocado as needed. Place the sauce in a bowl and leave it aside until the tacos are ready to be assembled.

Preheat your grill to medium-high. Drain the marinade off the steak. Throw away the marinade. Grill the steak for 4 to 6 minutes per side until medium rare. Place the steak on a chopping board and let aside for 10 minutes to rest. Using a large, sharp knife, thinly slice the steak against the grain.

Fill each tortilla with a couple of steak slices, 1 tablespoon chimichurri sauce, 14 cup lettuce, 1 tablespoon cheese, and 1 tablespoon salsa to assemble the tacos. Serve right away.

GLUTEN-FREE ADAPTABLE Choose gluten-free salsa and corn tortillas.

DAIRY-FREE AND ADAPTABLE Omit the cheese.

TIPS To warm flour tortillas, wrap a stack of three at a time in moist paper towels and microwave for 25 seconds, or until softened. Wrap them in foil with a few drops of water and heat them in the oven at 350°F for 10 to 15 minutes, until warm and pliable.

In a small pan, heat 13 cup vegetable oil over medium heat to fry corn tortillas. One at a time, fry the tortillas for about 10 seconds on each side. Place the tortillas on paper towels to drain, with a paper towel between each one.

Flank steak is most tender when it’s served as medium rare. When you poke the steak with your finger while it’s still raw, it’ll feel squishy. It will harden up while it cooks, so poke it again now and then. You don’t want it to become too firm, or the meat will become overcooked and tough. When it reaches 135°F on an instant-read thermometer, remove it off the grill.

If you want to serve steak instead of tacos, cook and slice the steak as directed, then top it with the avocado-chimichurri sauce.

lemonade with strawberries

Serves 4 people 15 minute prep time plus cooling/chilling time 5 minutes to prepare

My son used to have a lemonade stand. Serving freshly squeezed lemonade and home-baked cookies, he and his companion made approximately $50. I'm very sure we would have broken even if we had tallied up how much it truly cost to buy all of those ingredients. Regardless, because they worked so hard, I let them keep the money. They'll have to serve this strawberry version next time, which is likely to be even more popular.

1 tablespoon lemon zest, grated (see Tips)

1 cup lemon juice, freshly squeezed

2 cups simple syrup, thin (see Tips)

2 cups fresh strawberries, sliced

ice 2 cups sparkling water

Optional garnish: mint sprigs

Optional garnish: more sliced strawberries

In the cooled simple syrup, combine the lemon zest and lemon juice.

Puree the strawberries with 12 cup simple syrup in a blender. Combine the pureed strawberries and the remaining simple syrup in a medium mixing bowl. Pour the mixture into a pitcher via a fine sieve. Chill the mixture completely before serving.

Add the sparkling water to the pitcher when you're ready to serve the lemonade. Pour into glasses filled with ice. If preferred, garnish with a sprig of mint and sliced strawberries.

TIPS Before you squeeze the juice from your lemons, zest them.

Bring 2 cups water and 1 cup granulated white sugar to a boil in a small saucepan to make thin simple syrup. Reduce the heat to low and continue to stir until the sugar has completely dissolved. Remove the pan from the heat and set it aside to cool. Prepare and chill the simple syrup up to several days ahead of time.

This recipe is simple to duplicate or quadruple.

Chapter Six

Raspberry lemonade can be made by substituting raspberries for the strawberries.

To make a drink, add a splash of vodka to each individual serving.

Chapter Seven

sun tea from southern California

Approximately 8 servings Time to prepare: 4 hours + chill time 5 minutes to prepare

We don't have the same searing heat in Southern California as the nice Southern states. One summer, I travelled through those states. I adored the people, marvelled at the breathtaking environment, and ate some of the greatest food I'd ever tasted. But the oppressive heat, which they endure for days on end—oh my! It's quite harsh. We get summer heat in SoCal as too, but it is a little pleasant because there is no humidity. My refrigerator is always stocked with iced tea to keep us cool. My favourite is this gently sweetened tea.

7 cups water 2 large lemons' juice

4 tea bags (Earl Grey, English breakfast or original)

1 cup fresh mint leaves, loosely packed

1 cup simple syrup, thin (see Tips)

Ice

Optional extra mint leaves for garnish

Combine the 7 cups water and lemon juice in a big pitcher. Place the tea bags and mint leaves in the pitcher and cover with plastic wrap. For solar brewing, place the pitcher in the sun for 4 to 6 hours.

Remove the tea bags from the pitcher and drain the tea into another pitcher using a strainer. Remove and discard the mint leaves. Simply pour in the simple syrup. Refrigerate until thoroughly cooled, stirring occasionally. Tea should be served in large glasses with ice. If preferred, garnish each glass with a mint leaf.

TIPS To make thin simple syrup, boil 1 cup water and 12 cup granulated white sugar in a small saucepan. Reduce the heat to low and continue to stir until the sugar has completely dissolved. Remove the pan from the heat and set it aside to cool.

For a stronger, weaker, or sweeter taste, alter the amounts of tea, water, and sugar.

Leave out the syrup and add an extra cup of water to the pitcher for sun brewing if you don't want this to be a sweet tea. As desired, add sweetener to individual glasses.

Chapter Eight

Select flavoured tea. Orange-spice, cranberry, lemon-ginger, or your favourite are all good options.

Chapter Nine

limeade with cherries

Serves 4 to 6 people 20-minute prep time 5 minutes to prepare

My first Cherry Limeade was unforgettable. In the midst of summer, I was in Dallas visiting friends. That July, Dallas was hotter than any other place I'd ever been. One day, we stopped at a Sonic Drive-In for lunch, and I noticed Cherry Limeade on the menu. It sounded like a delightful drink that would be just refreshing on such a hot day. That's when my Cherry Limeade infatuation began. I took one and then took another. Before we left Dallas, I made numerous excuses to return to Sonic, and now I make my own Cherry Limeade at home. If you're serving a large group, double or triple the recipe.

1 cup simple syrup, thick (see Tips)

4–6 cups club soda, cold

1 cup lime juice, freshly squeezed

12 cup cherry maraschino juice

12 cup cherries maraschino

Ice

wedges of lime

Combine the simple syrup, 4 cups club soda, lime juice, cherry juice, and cherries in a pitcher. Taste after stirring. Add an additional 1 to 2 cups club soda if it's too sweet for your liking. Pour it into ice-filled glasses if it tastes good, being sure to get a few cherries in each glass. Serve with lime slices for garnish.

ADAPTABLE WITHOUT GLUTEN Make sure the maraschino cherries you use are gluten-free.

TIP Bring 1 cup water and 1 cup granulated white sugar to a boil in a small saucepan to make thick simple syrup. Reduce the heat to low and continue to stir until the sugar has completely dissolved. Remove the pan from the heat and set it aside to cool.

MAKE-AHEAD SUGGESTIONS Prepare and chill the simple syrup up to several days ahead of time.

Chapter Ten

This recipe also yields delicious basic limeade. Simply omit the cherries and juice and serve with lime slices as a garnish.

Chapter Eleven

temple, Shirley

Approximately 1 drink 5 minute prep time

This nonalcoholic childhood favourite was always one of my favourites, although we never made it at home. When I was a youngster, my father would order me a Shirley Temple before I could even say what I wanted. The simple shimmer, the pink tint, and the taste of a maraschino cherry combine to make this cocktail enticing. I make Shirley Temples at home for my son on special occasions. They're simple to make, and the youngsters believe they're a delight.

1 cup cubes of ice

1 lemon-lime soda can (7-Up or Sprite) a smidgeon of grenadine

1 cherry maraschino

Fill a glass with the ice cubes. Add the soda and grenadine to taste. Serve with a maraschino cherry as a garnish.

ADAPTABLE WITHOUT GLUTEN Use gluten-free brands of Coke, grenadine, and maraschino cherries.

TIP Drinking Shirley Temples using a straw is the most enjoyable.

Chapter Twelve

For those who enjoy maraschino cherries, go ahead and add more.

Chapter Thirteen

the finest sangria made with red wine

Approximately 6 servings 20-minute prep time

This recipe is referred regarded as "the best" because it is indeed the best. Sangria should not be sickeningly sweet, and this version is just right. It should be brimming with juicy, vibrant fruits like lemons, oranges, and limes. Grapes are also used in this sangria because they are a convenient fruit to eat while sipping. The addition of lemon juice and a small amount of club soda helps to balance out the flavours, resulting in a full-bodied drink with a light alcohol taste.

1 red wine bottle (750 mL) (see Tips)

a quarter-cup of orange juice

12 cup thick simple syrup + more sugar to taste (see Tips)

14 cup bourbon

14 cup liqueur orange (such as Grand Marnier)

1 tablespoon lemon juice, freshly squeezed

2 cups grapes (red and/or green)

1 finely sliced medium lemon

1 thinly sliced medium orange

1 finely sliced medium lime

10 oz. club soda, chilled

Combine all ingredients in a big pitcher or glass bowl (except the club soda). Allow at least 8 hours, but preferably 24 hours, for the sangria to marinate. Stir in the club soda right before serving. Serve the sangria in glasses with a ladle of fruit on the side.

This recipe does not require expensive wine. Use a dry wine such as Rioja or Syrah for this.

To make thick simple syrup, put 12 cup water and 12 cup granulated white sugar to a boil in a small pot. Reduce the heat to low and continue to stir until the sugar has completely dissolved. Remove the pan from the heat and set it aside to cool.

Chapter Fourteen

Add strawberries and/or red or green apple slices to this Sangria to change it up.

Pomegranate juice should be added to the mix.

Chapter Fifteen

Sangria with raspberry and peach lemonade

Approximately 8 servings 15-minute prep time

When it comes to happy hour, wine is always my drink of choice. When five o'clock rolls around, whether it's winter or summer, I enjoy a glass of ice-cold white wine. When fruit is at its peak in the summer, and I can't get enough of the luscious peaches and red ripe raspberries, I like to make fruity sangria instead of white wine. This recipe is especially refreshing in the summer since it includes lemonade.

1 750 mL bottle of dry white wine (Sauvignon Blanc or Pinot Grigio)

2 lemonade cups

limoncello (34 cup)

13 cup simple syrup, thick (see Tips)

1 cup fresh peaches, peeled, pitted, and sliced

1 cup raspberries or strawberries, fresh

1 finely sliced lemon

3 cups club soda, chilled

Combine all ingredients in a big pitcher or glass bowl (except club soda). Allow at least 8 hours, but preferably 24 hours, for the sangria to marinate. Stir in the club soda right before serving. Serve the sangria in glasses with a ladle of fruit on the side.

TIP To make thick simple syrup, put 13 cup water and 13 cup granulated white sugar to a boil in a small pot. Reduce the heat to low and continue to stir until the sugar has completely dissolved. Remove the pan from the heat and set it aside to cool.

Chapter Sixteen

Use rose wine and pink lemonade to make a lovely pink sangria.

Chapter Seventeen

pomegranate sparkling party punch

Serves 16 people 15-minute prep time

When I was younger, my mother had a Christmas cocktail party every year. Mom's coworkers and the entire neighbourhood descended on our humble abode to eat her famous stuffed mushrooms and excessive gallons of party punch. Mom always added an ice ring with maraschino cherries floating inside, so I'll never forget that punch. Before the visitors arrived, I made a game of swirling it about with the ladle. Although this is not Mom's party punch, it is equally popular. A tasty, effervescent drink made with pomegranate juice and ginger ale, white wine, vodka, and lemonade.

2 750 mL bottles of dry white wine (see Tip)

pomegranate juice, 2 cups

1 quart vodka

1 frozen lemonade concentrate 12-ounce can

For garnish, use pomegranate seeds, sliced lemons, and sliced oranges (as desired)

1 bottle ginger ale (2 litres)

Combine all ingredients in a big pitcher or basin (except ginger ale). Chill for several hours or overnight with chosen fruit toppings. Just before serving, add the ginger ale.

ADAPTABLE WITHOUT GLUTEN Use gluten-free lemonade concentrate and ginger ale brands.

TIP This recipe does not necessitate the purchase of pricey wine. A nice dry wine (such as Sauvignon Blanc or Pinot Grigio) at a reasonable price is ideal.

You may easily vary the flavour of this punch by replacing the pomegranate juice with another juice flavour.

Chapter Eighteen

tequila blueberry-pineapple punch

Approximately 8 servings Time to Prepare: 25 minutes

This will go down in history. My buddy Libbie was hosting a sort of get-together for some of our mutual friends who were moving. I came at Libbie's house early in the day to help with the preparation of some of the party's food and beverages. One of those drinks was this Tequila Punch with floating pineapple pieces and juicy blueberries. I arrived at the party early that night, eager to test it, only to discover that the punch had already been consumed. The first guests poured themselves a glass of punch, sipped it swiftly, and then poured another. The good news, I suppose, is that the punch has been designated a major favourite.

12 cup simple syrup, thick (see Tips)

12 cup lime juice, freshly squeezed

1 blueberry cup

34 cup fresh mint leaves, lightly packed

3 cups tequila silver (see Tips)

pineapple juice, 3 cups

12 cup pineapple slices (canned or fresh)

ice, crushed

Optional extra mint leaves for garnish

Optional garnish: fresh pineapple wedges

Combine the simple syrup, lime juice, blueberries, and mint in a large pitcher or punch bowl. With a wooden spoon, gently muddle everything together, mashing the blueberries and mint in the pitcher's bottom. Combine the tequila, pineapple juice, and pineapple chunks in a mixing glass. Before serving, chill for at least 4 hours. Over crushed ice, serve. If desired, garnish with mint leaves and/or pineapple wedges.

ADAPTABLE WITHOUT GLUTEN Use pineapple and juice brands that are known to be gluten-free.

TIPS To make thick simple syrup, put 12 cup water and 12 cup granulated white sugar to a boil in a small pot. Reduce the heat to low and continue to stir until the sugar has completely dissolved. Remove the pan from the heat and set it aside to cool.

Silver tequila is a clear spirit that is best used in cocktails with fruit. Gold tequila has a caramel flavour and is sweet and silky. It's best used for shots and margaritas.

Serve this cocktail in mason jars for a unique presentation.

mojito (orange-basil)

Serves 4 people Time to Prepare: 10 minutes

I tried this cocktail once while lounging poolside in Vegas, and I was so taken with it that I wanted to recreate it at home. If you've had a mojito before, you'll know that drink normally contains mint and lime juice. I just change basil for fresh mint and fresh orange juice for lime in the Orange-Basil Mojito. This makes for a truly unusual and delicious cocktail when muddled together and combined with rum and club soda.

1 cup orange juice, freshly squeezed

12 cup simple syrup, thick (see Tips)

10 big basil leaves, stems trimmed and thrown away

1 cup rum blanc

1 cup club soda

ice, crushed

Garnish with orange slices

For garnish, add more basil leaves.

Combine the orange juice, simple syrup, and basil in a medium pitcher. Crush the basil leaves in the bottom of the pitcher using a wooden spoon or a muddler. Combine the rum and club soda in a mixing glass. Serve over crushed ice in separate glasses right away. Serve with fresh basil and orange slices as garnish.

TIP To make thick simple syrup, put 12 cup water and 12 cup granulated white sugar to a boil in a small pot. Reduce the heat to low and continue to stir until the sugar has completely dissolved. Remove the pan from the heat and set it aside to cool.

Make a Strawberry-Basil Mojito with this cocktail. 14 cup freshly squeezed lime juice in place of orange juice, plus 112 cup cut strawberries Combine the basil, simple syrup, lime juice, and strawberries in a muddle. Combine the rum and 2 cups club soda in a mixing glass.

Chapter Nineteen

margaritas with mango

Approximately 6 drinks 15-minute prep time

I'm just going to admit it right now. I'm not a margarita drinker in the traditional sense. The salt has never appealed to me, the tequila is always too strong, and the flavour is just not for me. When I add strawberries, blueberries, peaches, or mango to a margarita, though, my story soon changes. I suppose there's something about sweetening a drink that makes it more enticing and desirable. Mango is one of my favourite flavours in a margarita, and this is one that I will cheerfully devour.

Ice

1 mango, sliced (fresh or frozen)

1 frozen limeade concentrate, 6 oz.

mango nectar, 6 oz (see Tips)

tequila, 4 oz.

3 oz Cointreau or triple sec

Optional: 2 ounces Grand Marnier Margarita salt

Optional garnish: lime wedges

Half-fill a blender with ice. In a blender, combine the mango, limeade concentrate, mango nectar, tequila, triple sec, and Grand Marnier. Blend until completely smooth (about 1 minute). Dip the rims of 6 glasses in water or mango nectar and then, if preferred, in salt. Serve the margaritas in the glasses with lime wedges on the side, if preferred.

ADAPTABLE WITHOUT GLUTEN Make sure the limeade and mango nectar you use are gluten-free.

TIP Mango nectar is commonly found in the bottled juice section of your supermarket.

This cocktail can be served “on the rocks” as well. Place the ice in the glasses instead of the mixer, and pour the blended cocktail over the ice.

Chapter Twenty

baked brie with a peach-gingered sauce

Approximately 8 servings 20-minute prep time Time to prepare: 20 minutes

One of my favourite appetisers to see on a client's list while I worked as a caterer in college was baked Brie. We bought these massive Brie rounds and carefully warmed them in enormous chafing pans. They were simply topped with almonds and dried cranberries. I'd wait as guests dipped baguette pieces into the hot, melted Brie, hoping there would be enough for me to try. This Brie is likewise hot and melted, and it's served with a sweet, gingery peach sauce, making it even more enticing than the Brie I recall.

1 cup peeled, pitted, and diced peaches (fresh, frozen, or canned)

14 cup light brown sugar, packed

2 tablespoons shallots, finely chopped

2 tbsp. apple cider vinegar

12 teaspoons cornstarch

12 teaspoon ground ginger (1 tablespoon grated fresh ginger)

1 cinnamon stick

1 teaspoon of salt

1 round Brie cheese (8 oz) (see Tips)

For serving, use baguette slices or crackers.

Combine all of the ingredients in a large pot (except cheese and baguette). Bring the mixture to a boil over medium heat and cook for 3 to 5 minutes, or until the peaches are softened. Remove the cinnamon stick and discard. While you prepare the cheese, leave the peach sauce at room temperature, covered.

Preheat the oven to 300 degrees Fahrenheit. Place the cheese in a pie plate or another oven-safe serving dish of similar size. Cut all the way around the rind at the top edge of the cheese with a sharp knife (don't remove the rind). Bake for 15 minutes, or until soft and melted cheese. To remove the rind, carefully cut under the top of the cheese (under the rind) using a sharp knife. Throw away the rind. On top of the cheese, pour the peach sauce. Serve with baguette pieces right away.

ADAPTABLE WITHOUT GLUTEN Instead of baguette pieces, serve with gluten-free crackers.

TIP Large warehouse stores, as well as some conventional grocery stores and specialty markets, frequently stock a nice-size round Brie.

MAKE-AHEAD SUGGESTIONS Make the peach sauce up to one day ahead of time. Refrigerate it well covered. Before serving, warm it in a medium saucepan over low heat.

Fresh blueberries can be used instead of peaches.

Chapter Twenty-one

dip with buffalo chicken

Serves 12 people 20-minute prep time 30 minutes to prepare

This dip, which is inspired by the iconic combo of buffalo wings, celery, and blue cheese dressing, combines all of those fantastic things into one. It's the kind of dip you'd serve at a sports-themed party or any other gathering when males congregate around the food table. Women will undoubtedly like this, as well.

1 cup cooked shredded chicken

34 cup Original Frank's RedHotTM Cayenne Pepper Sauce

1 8-ounce cream cheese package (see Tips)

1 box blue cheese crumbles, 5 oz

1 cup celery, finely chopped

1 cup cheddar-jack cheese, shredded (blended cheddar and Monterey Jack cheeses)

34 cup tiny cherry or pear tomatoes, halved

12 cup green onion, chopped Serve with celery sticks and tortilla chips.

Preheat the oven to 350 degrees Fahrenheit. Using nonstick spray, coat an 8-inch square pan.

Combine the chicken and cayenne pepper sauce in a medium mixing basin. Pour the mixture into the prepared pan's bottom.

Melt the cream cheese in a small saucepan over medium heat. Mix until smooth, then stir in the blue cheese crumbles until thoroughly blended. Remove the chicken from the heat and spread the cheese mixture over it. Add the celery to the top.

Bake for 20 minutes, uncovered. Remove the skillet from the oven and sprinkle the cheddar-Jack cheese over the hot dip. Return to the oven for another 10 minutes, or until the cheese has melted. Before serving, remove the dip from the oven and top with the cherry tomatoes and green onion. Serve with tortilla chips and celery sticks.

TIPS You can use lower-fat cream cheese in this recipe, but don't use low-fat cheese for the topping because it won't melt properly.

To make this dip even more vibrant, look for multicoloured cherry tomatoes.

If you can't get Frank's brand sauce, any type of Buffalo sauce will suffice.

Instead of ranch dressing, use a spicy barbecue sauce in this dip. It will change the flavour of the dip, but it will still be delicious!

Chapter Twenty-two

In a bread dish, serve a hot seafood dip.

Serves 12 people 30 minute prep time 1 hour and 45 minutes to prepare

When served in a bread bowl, clam chowder is delicious, so why not a seafood dip? The resulting bread chunks are available for dipping when the bread bowl is sliced out to make way for the dip, and as the bread chunks disappear, people appear to relish manhandling the bowl, pulling off bits to sink into this hot and creamy dip.

1 8-ounce container room temperature cream cheese

8 oz. soured cream

1 cup Parmesan cheese, freshly grated

1 cup celery, finely chopped

¼ cup beer

14 cup sweet onion, shredded

1 tablespoon horseradish, prepared

1 teaspoon of Worcestershire sauce

2 tablespoons lemon juice, freshly squeezed

1 tsp. chilli sauce

12 teaspoon salt (garlic)

a quarter teaspoon of salt

2 6.5-ounce minced clam cans, squeezed dry + 2 teaspoons retained juice

1 small shrimp can (drained and pressed dry)

1 round French or sourdough bread, 20 oz.

14 cup green onion, chopped

Optional baguette pieces for dipping

Preheat the oven to 300 degrees Fahrenheit. Using nonstick spray, coat an 8-inch square pan.

Whisk together the cream cheese and sour cream in a large mixing basin until smooth. Combine the Parmesan, celery, beer, onion, horseradish, Worcestershire sauce, lemon juice, spicy sauce, garlic salt, and salt in a mixing bowl. Stir in the clams and conserved clam liquid, as well as the shrimp. Cover the prepared dish with foil after scraping the creamy seafood mixture into it. 12 hours in the oven

Cut around the top edge of the bread with a serrated knife. Remove the top and chop it up into little pieces. To make a bowl, scoop out the bread. Tear the bread into bite-size pieces after it has been scooped out. Fill a sealed container or zip baggie with all of the bread pieces and the bowl. Place aside.

Remove the bread bowl from the oven and carefully spoon the dip into it. Before serving, place the bread dish on a baking sheet and return it to the oven for another 15 minutes. Place the bread bowl dip on a serving tray, top with the green onion, and serve immediately with the bread pieces and more baguette slices, if preferred.

TIP If preferred, 112 cup fresh clams and tiny shrimp can be substituted for the canned.

Make a luscious lobster dip with this. Instead of clams and shrimp, use 112 cups lobster meat.

Chapter Twenty-three

dip with caramelised onions

3 cup serving Time to Prepare: 25 minutes 30 minutes to prepare

When you're watching your favourite teams play on TV, nothing beats having a tub of store-bought onion dip by your side with a bag of your favourite potato chips, right? However, if you can substitute it with something that is homemade, sweet, delicious, and amazing, I guarantee you will never desire tub food again.

2 tablespoons extra virgin olive oil

3 cups sweet onion, finely diced

divided 34 teaspoon kosher salt

12 gallon sour cream

a quarter-cup of mayonnaise

12 teaspoon powdered garlic

a quarter teaspoon of white pepper

To taste, a dash of hot sauce (Tabasco or something similar).

Optional: 18 tsp red pepper flakes

Serve with sturdy potato chips.

Heat the olive oil in a large skillet over medium heat. Add the onion and a quarter teaspoon of salt to the pan. Cook, stirring occasionally, for about 30 minutes, or until the onion begins to caramelise and turn golden brown. Because you want the onions to brown, don't stir them frequently, but keep an eye on them to make sure they're not browning too quickly or burning, and adjust the heat as needed. Take the onions off the fire and let them cool.

Mix the remaining 12 teaspoon salt, sour cream, mayonnaise, garlic powder, white pepper, spicy sauce, and red pepper flakes in a medium mixing bowl, then add the cooled onions. Season to taste with extra garlic powder, salt, and/or spicy sauce, if preferred. Allow to chill until ready to serve. Serve with a stir. Serve alongside thick potato chips.

ADAPTABLE WITHOUT GLUTEN Make sure to use gluten-free mayonnaise and potato chips.

TIPS Make this dip a day ahead of time to allow the flavours to meld completely.

Use low-fat sour cream and low-fat mayonnaise to make this a lower-fat dip.

Instead of sweet onions, use red onions.

Add some chopped roasted red peppers to the mix.

dip with artichokes and bacon

Serves 12 people Time to Prepare: 25 minutes 45 minutes to prepare

A rich and creamy dip with artichoke hearts and crispy bacon pieces. It's one of those dips that's difficult to put down after just a few bites. Serve this appetiser on a day when you need warmth and comfort and you have a huge, hungry crowd waiting for you. It's excellent comfort food in general.

8 oz. cream cheese, cut into chunks

1 drained and finely chopped 14-ounce can artichoke hearts

1 cup drained and coarsely chopped roasted red peppers from a jar

1 pound mayonnaise

12 cup celery, finely diced

4 oz. crumbled Gorgonzola or blue cheese

white wine (13 cup)

1 big beaten egg

12 teaspoon powdered garlic

12 cup bacon, cooked and crumbled (about 8 slices; see Tips)

For serving, use pita chips or baguette slices.

Preheat the oven to 350 degrees Fahrenheit. Using nonstick spray, coat a 9-inch pie plate.

Melt the cream cheese in a small saucepan over low heat. Stir until completely smooth. In a large mixing bowl, scrape the melted cream cheese. Mix in the rest of the ingredients (except bacon and chips). Fill the pie plate halfway with the mixture. Bake for 25 minutes, covered in foil. Remove the foil and bake for another 25 minutes, or until the dip is bubbling and baked through. Add the bacon on the top. Serve with pita chips or baguette pieces right away.

ADAPTABLE WITHOUT GLUTEN Replace the Gorgonzola cheese with goat or feta cheese, and use gluten-free mayonnaise and bacon. With gluten-free crackers on the side.

ADAPTABLE TO VEGETARIANS Leave the bacon out.

TIP Cook your bacon in the oven for simple cleanup. Preheat the oven to 400 degrees Fahrenheit. Place a rack on top of a big, rimmed baking sheet lined with foil. Using nonstick spray, coat the rack. On the rack, arrange the bacon strips. Bake for 15 to 20 minutes, or until crisp. The length of time depends on how thick your bacon is.

Mix in a 10-ounce box of frozen spinach to make a spinach-artichoke dip (thawed and squeezed dry).

Chapter Twenty-four

Mediterranean spinach dip with layers

Serves 12 people Time to Prepare: 25 minutes

For many people, the ease of picking up a tub of store-bought hummus is all too familiar and comforting. With some carrots and a handful of chips for dipping, you've got yourself a no-fuss appetiser. However, if you want to go the additional mile and add a few minutes to your prep time, you'll have hummus and a lot more to give your visitors. This recipe mixes spinach dip with hummus, tomato, feta cheese, and Kalamata olives to make something a little different from the typical store-bought tub.

12 cup fresh spinach greens, packed

1 drained 5-ounce can of sliced water chestnuts

4 ounces room temperature cream cheese

sour cream (12 cup)

1 tablespoon lemon juice, freshly squeezed

12 teaspoon sodium chloride

1/8 teaspoon black pepper, freshly ground

10 ounces hummus (prepared) (store-bought is fine)

1 cup tomato, chopped

12 cup Kalamata olives, roughly chopped

12 cup feta cheese, crumbled

13 cup green onion, white and light green portions chopped

To serve, pita chips

Combine the spinach, water chestnuts, cream cheese, sour cream, lemon juice, salt, and pepper in a food processor. Pulse until the ingredients are thoroughly blended and pureed. Fill a 9-inch round or square serving dish halfway with purée (or something similar). To make the second layer of the dip, spoon the hummus on top of the spinach puree and smooth it out evenly. Add tomato, olives, and feta cheese to the second layer. On top, scatter the green onions. Allow to chill until ready to serve. Serve with dipping pita chips.

ADAPTABLE WITHOUT GLUTEN Make sure to use gluten-free hummus and Kalamata olives. With gluten-free crackers on the side.

TIP This dip can be made up to 4 hours ahead of time. Refrigerate until ready to serve, covered lightly with plastic wrap.

Layer cucumber finely sliced between the layers.

Use roasted garlic or roasted red pepper hummus instead of plain hummus.

Chapter Twenty-five

7-layer mexican dip from Southern California

Makes one 9 x 13-inch dip pan 30 minute prep time 18 minutes to prepare

The idea of a seven-layer Mexican dip has been around for a long time. Most grocery stores now sell the easy-to-make dip already layered in a plastic tub. The plastic tub version is unpleasant to me because of the congealed sour cream and faux guacamole. Making your own layer dip is actually fairly simple. Crispy bacon, maize, crumbled Mexican Cojita cheese, and, of course, authentic guacamole have been added to the basic version. It's simple to make, and I guarantee it'll taste better than a plastic tub dip.

10 bacon slices

3 pitted, peeled, and cored avocados

a quarter-cup of sour cream, split

1 tablespoon lime juice, freshly squeezed

To taste, season with salt and freshly ground black pepper.

1 large cob of corn, shucked, rinsed, and dried

1 refried bean can (30 ounces)

2 cups Roma tomato, chopped (about 4 large)

1 cup Cojita cheese, crumbled (see Tips)

Dippable tortilla chips

In the oven, cook the bacon (see Tips). Prepare the rest of the dip while the bacon is cooking.

In a medium bowl, mash the avocados and whisk in 14 cup of sour cream and the lime juice to make a simple guacamole. To taste, season the guacamole with salt and pepper.

Remove the kernels off the cob of corn (see Tips).

To make the dip, lightly coat a 9 x 13-inch baking dish with nonstick spray. In the bottom of the dish, spread the refried beans. Spread the remaining 112 cup sour cream evenly over the top. Spread the guacamole on top of the sour cream and spread it gently to the borders to cover it. Toss the tomato on top. Over the tomato, crumble the bacon. Corn and cheese should be layered. Refrigerate the dip until ready to serve by wrapping it in plastic wrap. Toss with tortilla chips before serving.

ADAPTABLE WITHOUT GLUTEN Make sure to use gluten-free bacon, refried beans, and tortilla chips.

ADAPTABLE TO VEGETARIANS Leave the bacon out.

TIPS Cook your bacon in the oven for simple cleanup. Preheat the oven to 400 degrees Fahrenheit. Place a rack on top of a big, rimmed baking sheet lined with foil. Using nonstick spray, coat the rack. On the rack, arrange the bacon strips. Bake for 15 to 20 minutes, or until crisp. The length of time depends on how thick your bacon is.

Cut a short slice off the end of the cob to produce a flat surface for cutting the corn kernels off the cob. Place the flat end of the corn in the centre of a bowl and hold it there. With a sharp knife, cut along the sides of the cob, and the corn kernels will collect inside the bowl.

Cojita cheese is a Mexican crumbly cheese. It's frequently found in your market's speciality cheese area. Feta cheese can be used instead.

This dip can be made up to 2 hours ahead of time.

More layers can be added, such as fresh chopped cilantro, black olives, or chopped green onions.

Chapter Twenty-six

veggie dip (curry-dill)

3 cup serving 15 minute prep time plus chill time

I have a curry-dill dip recipe stuck in my head for some inexplicable reason. When my mother offered fresh veggies as an appetiser to guests, she made a simple herbed curry and dill dip to accompany them. As a result, I always think of curry as the foundation for a vegetable dip. This recipe is similar to Mom's dip, except it adds fresh herbs and spinach, as well as a creamier texture. The curry flavour is mild, but more can be added if desired.

1 tablespoon mayonnaise

1 gallon sour cream

1 cup fresh spinach leaves, packed

4 oz. goat cheese crumbles

2 tablespoons fresh parsley, chopped

1 tablespoon fresh dill, chopped

curry powder (1 teaspoon)

12 teaspoon salt (celery)

12 teaspoon powdered onion

Optional garnish: 1 tablespoon chopped fresh chives

a variety of dipping vegetables (see Tips)

Combine all of the ingredients (except the chives and dipping veggies) in a food processor and mix until smooth. Place in the refrigerator until ready to serve. Transfer the dip to a serving bowl and top with chives, if desired, before serving. Serve alongside a variety of vegetables.

ADAPTABLE WITHOUT GLUTEN Make sure to use a gluten-free mayonnaise.

TIPS Cucumber slices, broccoli, zucchini, radish, cauliflower, cherry or pear tomatoes, carrots, and celery are also good dipping veggies.

This dip can be made up to two days ahead of time.

If you don't have a food processor or like a more streamlined herb-only dip, leave off the spinach.

1 teaspoon lemon juice, freshly squeezed

Chapter Twenty-seven

salsa strawberry-avocado

Serves 212 cups salsa 15-minute prep time

The little things in life can sometimes fill your stomach and make you smile. One of those things is this incredibly simple fruit salsa. It's best made when strawberries are extremely ripe and sweet, and all you need are a few chips for scooping.

1 cup fresh strawberries, finely diced

1 avocado, finely diced (1 medium)

12 cup sweet onion, coarsely chopped

2 tablespoons lime juice, freshly squeezed

2 tablespoons jalapeo, finely chopped (seeds and ribs removed)

Dippable tortilla chips

In a medium mixing dish, combine all of the ingredients (except the tortilla chips). Serve with tortilla chips right away.

ADAPTABLE WITHOUT GLUTEN Make sure the tortilla chips you use are gluten-free.

TIP This is not a recipe that should be prepared ahead of time. When avocado is exposed to air, it begins to oxidise, which causes it to turn brown. The addition of lime juice slows but does not completely stop the oxidation process. Prepare the salsa ahead of time and serve immediately.

Avocado also goes well with other fruits. Strawberry can be replaced with peach, nectarine, or mango.

Chapter Twenty-eight

Mango-chipotle guacamole, sweet and smokin' hot

2 cup serving 20-minute prep time

I used to enter recipes in contests at the San Diego County Fair when I first became interested in cooking. My strawberry-coconut cheesecake won second place in the cheesecake competition one year. I was thrilled to learn that they were holding a guacamole competition a few years later. I've always considered myself a guacamole connoisseur, so I worked hard to perfect this recipe, which included chopped mango, chipotle, and bacon, with the goal of entering it in the Fair's contest. When I realised that I was no longer eligible to enter (as a food professional), my hopes of winning the ultimate prize were dashed. So instead, I'm sharing it with my cookbook readers. So, what are your thoughts on prize-winning potential?

2 medium avocados, fully ripe (see Tips)

12 medium lime (distributed)

2 tblsp. soured cream

12 teaspoon sauce + 1 teaspoon minced chipotle chiles in adobo sauce, seeds removed (see Tips)

34 cup fresh mango, diced, divided

3 bacon slices, cooked till crisp and crumbly, divided

3 tablespoons salsa (fresh)

To taste, season with salt and freshly ground black pepper.

To serve, tortilla chips and/or jicama slices

Mash the avocado with a fork in a medium bowl, leaving some pieces. On top, squeeze the juice from 14 limes. Combine the sour cream, chipotles, and sauce in a mixing bowl. Stir until everything is well blended. 12 cup mango, 2 pieces crumbled bacon, and salsa in a mixing bowl Season to taste with salt and pepper. Drizzle the remaining 14 teaspoons of lime juice over the guacamole. Finish with the leftover bacon crumbles and mango.

Serve with tortilla chips and/or jicama slices right away (or soon). If you need to keep the guacamole in the fridge for an hour or two before serving, throw a piece of plastic wrap on top and press it against the guacamole. This will keep air out and keep your guacamole from going brown.

ADAPTABLE WITHOUT GLUTEN Choose gluten-free bacon, chipotles in adobo, and tortilla chips.

ADAPTABLE DAIRY-FREE Leave the sour cream out.

ADAPTABLE TO VEGETARIANS Leave the bacon out.

TIPS Hold an avocado in your hand and lightly press it to see if it's ripe. When you press down on a properly ripe avocado, it has a little give to it. It's too ripe if it's easy to squash. It's overly ripe if there are any squishy (or hollow) patches. If you can't find avocados that are ready to eat because they aren't quite ripe, bring them home and leave them on your counter for a day or two. To hasten the ripening process, place them in a paper bag.

Chipotle peppers in adobo sauce are canned and should be found in the Latin-American products department of your supermarket. You'll have plenty of leftover chipotles in adobo if you open a new can. They freeze beautifully. Simply spoon a chipotle pepper and some sauce into individual zip baggies and freeze them. When you need them again, simply let them thaw.

Fresh salsa is frequently accessible in the deli department of your supermarket, along with other chilled Latin-American foods.

This dish only requires basic bacon. Use applewood smoked bacon if you can locate it; it has a great, smoky flavour. Some grocery stores and specialty marketplaces carry the applewood variety.

Add more chipotle sauce to make this dip extra spicy. Add a small amount at a time until you reach the desired level of spice.

goat cheese, pear, and caramelised shallots pizzette

Prep Time: 35 minutes Cook Time: 25 minutes Yield: 18 appetisers

In the world of cuisine, there is an unwritten law that caramelising everything makes it taste better. Do you know what this rule is? These easy little pizza appetisers are topped with goat cheese, pear, and fresh thyme before being topped with a liberal sprinkling of caramelised shallots to make them worthy of at least four bites. That unwritten rule is fantastic.

1 tablespoon olive oil + 2 tablespoons extra virgin olive oil, divided

6 medium peeled and thinly sliced shallots

1 tablespoon salt

pizza dough (1 pound) (see Tips)

1 pound goat cheese log

1 pear, ripe but not overripe, peeled and thinly sliced into 2-inch wedges

1 tablespoon thyme leaves, chopped

1 tablespoon olive oil, heated in a medium skillet over medium heat Add the shallots and season with salt. Reduce the heat to medium-low and simmer, stirring frequently, for 15 to 20 minutes, or until the shallots are tender and lightly browned. Place aside.

Preheat the oven to 475 degrees Fahrenheit. Use parchment paper or a Silpat mat to line a baking sheet.

Roll out the pizza dough to a thickness of 14 inches on a lightly floured board. Cut 18 rounds of dough using a 212 inch round biscuit cutter, rerolling as needed (see Tips). Brush the rounds lightly with the remaining 2 teaspoons olive oil and place them on the prepared baking sheet. Spread about 12 tbsp goat cheese on each circle, then top with two overlapping slices of pear. Bake for 8 to 10 minutes, or until golden brown on top.

Place each pizzette on a serving dish and top with 12 tablespoons caramelised shallots and a sprig of thyme.

TIPS Make your own pizza dough, buy prepared pizza dough at the store, or ask a pizza establishment to sell you a 1-pound dough ball.

If you don't have a biscuit cutter, use the top of a drinking glass with a diameter of about 212 inches.

Replace the shallots with sweet onions or red onions, increasing the cooking time to 20 to 25 minutes, and replace the goat cheese with soft, spreadable herb cheese.

zucchini with balsamic glaze and cheese-stuffed mushrooms

Makes 24 mushrooms; 35 minutes to prepare; 25 minutes to cook

I'm not sure why my son refuses to eat mushrooms. My mother's "renowned" stuffed mushrooms, which were simply mushrooms stuffed with mushroom bits and sausage, were something I grew up eating. They were so simple, but they worked, and they were always consumed very quickly after being taken out of the oven. I chose to go a different path with my recipe because sausage is utilised in so many stuffed mushroom recipes these days. These are packed with zucchini, onion, and Swiss cheese then marinated in balsamic vinegar. At a party, I think you'll discover that they're quite popular. But no matter what I do to mushrooms, I can't seem to get my own child to touch them. I guess that just means I'll be getting more of these.

MARINADE

balsamic vinegar, 3 teaspoons

12 teaspoons garlic, minced

12 tablespoons mustard (Dijon)

STUFFING AND MUSHROOMS

24 white mushrooms, medium to large (212-inch diameter), stems removed, cleaned, and dried

1 cup packed shredded zucchini (about 112 large zucchini), squeezed dry

12 cup Gruyère or Swiss cheese, grated

12 cup bread crumbs (Italian style)

13 cup sweet onion, coarsely chopped

14 teaspoon black pepper, freshly ground

heavy whipping cream, 2 to 3 teaspoons

1 tablespoon extra virgin olive oil

Optional: 2 tablespoons finely chopped flat-leaf parsley

Preheat the oven to 375 degrees Fahrenheit.

Whisk together the marinade ingredients in a small bowl.

In a 9 x 13-inch glass dish, arrange the mushrooms stem side up. 12 teaspoon marinade drizzled into each mushroom

To make the stuffing, combine the zucchini, cheese, bread crumbs, onion, and pepper in a medium mixing bowl.

2 tablespoons cream and 2 teaspoons olive oil, whisked together When a spoon is placed against the mixture, it should come together somewhat damp. Provide any residual marinade and, if necessary, another tablespoon of cream to add moisture.

Fill the mushroom cavities with the stuffing, slightly mounding it. Pour 3 tablespoons of water into the pan's bottom. Bake for 25 to 30 minutes, or until the mushrooms are soft and the filling is hot and brown on top. If preferred, top the mushrooms with flat-leaf parsley and serve right away.

GLUTEN-FREE ADAPTABLE Use a gluten-free Dijon mustard. Replace the usual bread crumbs with gluten-free bread crumbs.

TIP Stuffed mushrooms are best served immediately after baking. Serve them to your guests on a tray with toothpicks and napkins, and distribute them immediately while they are still warm.

For the Swiss/Gruyère, use 1 cup shredded Parmesan or provolone.

The sensitive sections of the mushroom stems should be chopped and included in the filling.

cucumber rounds topped with cured salmon

Makes 30 appetisers; 40 minutes to prepare

When you need a quick and exquisite appetiser, thank heavens for smoked salmon. It comes in a small packet in your market, ready to serve without the need for cooking, and it's a lovely addition to your appetiser display. Cucumber slices are coated with a creamy caper and horseradish cheese, then topped with smoked salmon and fresh dill in this recipe.

1 pound sour cream

3 ounces room temperature cream cheese

2 teaspoons capers, chopped

1 tablespoon horseradish, prepared

To taste, season with salt and freshly ground black pepper.

1 big English hothouse cucumber, cut into thirty 14-inch slices crosswise

smoked salmon, 12 pound, sliced into 112-inch chunks

30 12-inch dill pieces

Stir together the sour cream, cream cheese, capers, and horseradish in a medium mixing bowl until smooth. Season to taste with salt and pepper.

Fill each cucumber slice with a heaping teaspoon of the cheese mixture. Garnish with a slice of dill and a folded-over chunk of salmon on top of the cheese. Before serving, chill for up to 2 hours.

ADAPTABLE TO GLUTEN-FREE INGREDIENTS Use gluten-free horseradish and smoked salmon brands.

QUICK AND EASY TIP: In place of the cream cheese mixture, get a soft herb tub cheese.

Serve this appetiser on top of square-shaped cocktail bread, cucumber and all.

bruschetta with nectarine

Makes 24 appetisers; 30 minutes to prepare; 10 minutes to cook

Sweet nectarines are paired with the acidic flavour of feta cheese to form a wonderful summer treat in this unique spin on a no-tomato bruschetta. When nectarines are sweet and ripe, they're best. This is an appetiser that even the kids will like.

2 pitted and finely diced medium ripe nectarines (about 1 cup)

12 medium diced red bell pepper (approximately 23 cup)

3 green onions, chopped (just the white parts)

3 tblsp. extra virgin olive oil, divided

1 tablespoon lime juice, freshly squeezed

1 teaspoon Serrano chile, minced

Baguette with 24 thin slices

34 cup feta cheese, crumbled

Preheat the oven to 350°F and position the rack in the centre.

Toss the nectarines, bell pepper, onions, 1 tablespoon olive oil, lime juice, and chile in a medium bowl gently. Place aside.

On a baking sheet, arrange the baguette slices. Drizzle the remaining 2 tablespoons olive oil over the bread. 3 to 5 minutes in the oven, until the baguette slices are lightly toasted (watch closely so they don't overbrown or burn).

Remove the bread from the oven and spread a dollop of the nectarine mixture on each piece. On top, sprinkle the cheese. Return the baking sheet to the oven and bake the bruschetta for another 3 to 5 minutes, or until they are well heated. Serve right away.

GLUTEN-FREE ADAPTABLE Instead of baguette pieces, serve the sweet nectarine mixture over gluten-free crackers.

DAIRY-FREE AND ADAPTABLE Omit the cheese.

TIPS Cut the baguette on a slight diagonal to get somewhat larger, more beautiful bread slices.

This dish is also delicious cold, served on toasted baguette pieces.

Try substituting peaches or sweet plums for nectarines, and goat cheese for feta cheese. Toss in some chopped prosciutto.

Pinwheels of puff pastry with spinach, sun-dried tomato, and prosciutto

Preparation Time: 15 minutes + chilling/freezing time Cooking Time: 20 minutes

This pinwheel snack is also very easy to make. You don't need to be a TV chef to make them, but everyone always says they're festive and amazing. They're a terrific make-ahead alternative because you can freeze them and use them whenever you want.

1 17.3-ounce puff pastry package (2 sheets)

1 frozen 10-ounce container chopped spinach, thawed and squeezed dry

12 cup sun-dried tomatoes, chopped (see Tips)

1 pound mayonnaise

12 cup Asiago or Parmesan cheese, freshly grated

1 teaspoon powdered onion

1 teaspoon powdered garlic

14 teaspoon black pepper, freshly ground

5 oz. prosciutto thinly sliced

1 large beaten egg, combined with 1 tablespoon water

Puff pastry should be defrosted and simple to unroll after 30 minutes at room temperature.

In a medium mixing bowl, combine the spinach, sun-dried tomatoes, mayonnaise, cheese, onion powder, garlic powder, and pepper to make the filling. Refrigerate until ready to use, covered.

Unfold 1 sheet of puff pastry and arrange it with the long side facing you on a lightly floured board. Half of the spinach mixture should be spread equally across the pastry sheet, with a 12-inch border around the perimeter. Half of the prosciutto slices should be placed on top of the spinach. Roll up the pastry from the long side facing you, pressing to seal the seam. Wrap plastic wrap around the log. Repeat with the rest of the pastry, spinach mixture, and prosciutto. Freeze the rolled-up pastry logs for 45 minutes, or until firm but not frozen.

Preheat the oven to 400 degrees Fahrenheit. Place the pastry logs on two baking sheets, leaving 112 inches between each pinwheel, and cut into 12-inch thick slices. Apply egg wash to each pinwheel. Preheat oven to 200°F and bake for 20–25 minutes, or until golden brown. Warm or at room temperature is fine.

TIPS Rehydrate dried tomatoes in boiling water until softened, or use sun-dried tomatoes packed in oil (drain and pat dry) (drain and pat dry).

These appetisers can be cut, frozen on baking sheets, packaged, and stored in the freezer for up to three months. As needed, remove the slices from the freezer and bake.

Layer 2 tablespoons honey mustard, 5 ounces thinly sliced prosciutto, and 34 cup shredded Parmesan cheese in a fresh variation of a puff pastry pinwheel.

fig, blue cheese, and honeyed walnuts filled endive

Prep Time: 40 minutes Cook Time: 10 minutes Yield: 18 appetisers

Endive belongs to the chicory family, which includes radicchio and escarole. It's a vegetable that comes apart with little, crisp leaves that act as a natural resting spot for appetiser fillings. The leaves are filled with a blue cheese spread, dried figs, and toasted honeyed walnuts in this two-bite appetiser recipe.

12 cup walnuts, roughly chopped

112 teaspoons honey

3 oz. softened cream cheese

13 cup crumbled blue cheese

1 tbsp. soured cream

2 endive heads, leaves detached

9 figs (dry) sliced into thirds

Preheat the oven to 350 degrees Fahrenheit. Using nonstick spray, coat a baking sheet.

Combine the walnuts and honey in a small bowl. Sprinkle them on the baking sheet and bake for 10 minutes, stirring halfway through. Allow to cool after removing from the oven.

Cream together the cream cheese, blue cheese, and sour cream in a medium mixing basin until creamy.

Fill each endive leaf with 2 teaspoons of the cream cheese mixture. 1 fig slice and 1 teaspoon walnuts on top of each.

GLUTEN-FREE ADAPTABLE Use a fig brand that is known to be gluten-free, and replace the blue cheese with feta or goat cheese.

TIPS Use fresh figs instead of dried figs when they're in season.

This meal can be prepared 2 to 3 hours ahead of time. Place in the refrigerator until ready to serve.

Replace the walnuts with pecans, the blue cheese with goat cheese, and the figs with dried apricots.

Scallops in a creamy bacon-balsamic sauce (for two)

Prep Time: 15 minutes Cook Time: 10 minutes Yield: 2 serves

Recipes for two are ideal for a small snack before your romantic (or ho-hum, we've been married for a long time) supper. Scallops cook quickly and simply on the stove, making them an excellent appetiser option. You'll wish you didn't have to split them with a generous drizzle of balsamic cream sauce and a sprinkling of bacon.

2 tablespoons shallot, finely chopped

2 bacon pieces, finely chopped (see Tips)

4 scallops, big

12 tbsp garlic, minced

white wine, 2 teaspoons

14 cup heavy cream (whipped)

balsamic vinegar, 1 tbsp

14 cup tomato, seeded and sliced

Optional garnish: chopped fresh chives or flat-leaf parsley

Cook the shallot and bacon in a medium skillet over medium heat for 5 to 6 minutes, or until the shallots soften and brown and the bacon is crisp. Cook, stirring occasionally, until the scallops are gently browned below, 2 to 3 minutes. Cook for 30 seconds after adding the garlic. Add the wine to the pan after flipping the scallops. Cook until the wine has almost completely evaporated. Pour in the cream and the vinegar. Cook the scallops in the sauce for 2 to 3 minutes more, or until they are cooked through.

Place two scallops on each of two dishes and drizzle with balsamic cream sauce and 2 tablespoons tomato for serving. If desired, garnish with chives or parsley.

ADAPTABLE TO GLUTEN-FREE BACON Choose a gluten-free bacon brand.

TIP I prefer center-cut bacon for this dish since it yields more bacon with less fat.

Serve the scallops and sauce over hot cooked pasta to make this a one-person meal.

Shooters of chilled strawberry and coconut milk soup

Makes 10 soup shooters Time to prepare: 15 minutes plus marinating time

Chilled soup may appear to be a strange commodity, but it isn't. It's a fun and sophisticated appetiser to serve, but it's not difficult to make. Everything can be made in a blender, and the preparation time is short. Serve in little plastic cups or tall shot glasses with a small strawberry as a garnish and a sprinkling of toasted coconut on top. "Fun summer appetiser" is written all over this one. It will also appeal to children.

8 ounces washed and sliced strawberries

2 teaspoons white granulated sugar

1 tablespoon lime juice, freshly squeezed

1 cup canned coconut milk (low-fat)

garnish with additional small strawberries

14 cup toasted shaved coconut (for decoration) (optional; see Tips)

In a medium mixing dish, combine the strawberries, sugar, and lime juice. Allow 30 minutes for the mixture to marinade.

Combine the strawberries and coconut milk in a blender or food processor. Blend until completely smooth. If preferred, top with strawberries and toasted coconut in tiny serving glasses.

Preheat the oven to 350°F before toasting the coconut. Spread the coconut out on a rimmed baking sheet and bake for 4 to 6 minutes, or until golden (stirring halfway through). If you sweeten the coconut, it will brown faster, so keep an eye on it.

Make this a cocktail instead of an appetiser by adding white rum or coconut rum.

jalapeos filled with chorizo and cheese

Makes 20 appetisers; 30 minutes to prepare; 15 minutes to cook

My roommates and I used to go to several of the nice local places for happy hour when we were in college. Our goal was to assemble a cheap dinner from the "Happy Hour Appetizer Specials" menu, and then devour as many calories as humanly possible in one sitting. The infamous deep-fried jalapeo popper was one of the appetisers that contributed to that ultimately poor decision. I believe I'm still recovering from the long-term effects of those deep-fried appetisers on my thighs. My filled jalapeos dish isn't quite as sinister as those college snacks. They're baked instead of fried and packed with cheese deliciousness and a little chorizo mixed with corn tortilla crumbs.

10 medium jalapeo peppers, fresh

6 oz. cooked and crumbled pork chorizo

4 oz. softened cream cheese

12 cup crumbs from tortillas (see Tips)

12 cup extra sharp cheddar cheese, finely shredded

a quarter teaspoon of garlic powder

14 teaspoon powdered onion

1/8 teaspoon black pepper, freshly ground

14 cup fresh cilantro, chopped + extra sprigs for garnish

Preheat the oven to 400 degrees Fahrenheit.

Half the jalapeos lengthwise, leaving the stem on one half intact. Remove and discard the seeds and ribs (see Tips).

To make the filling, combine the chorizo and the remaining ingredients in a medium mixing dish (except cilantro). Fill each half of a jalapeo with the filling, slightly mounding it. On a baking sheet, arrange the stuffed jalapeos.

Bake for 15 to 20 minutes, or until the peppers have softened and the filling has heated through. Sprinkle the chopped cilantro over the jalapeos and place them on a serving plate. Serve immediately after garnishing the plate with cilantro sprigs.

GLUTEN-FREE ADAPTABLE Choose gluten-free chorizo and corn tortillas.

TIPS Handle the jalapeos with caution because they will leave a burning sensation on your hands. To avoid this from happening, use gloves when handling. Because the ribs and seeds of the pepper are the most fiery parts, eliminate them altogether.

To make 12 cup of crumbs, grind 2 corn tortillas in a food processor or blender. There's no need to buy something new. If you have older, semi-stale tortillas on hand, they'll work just well in the grinder.

Replace the chorizo with hot Italian sausage and the tortilla crumbs with bread crumbs.

sweet-and-sticky chicken wings

Preparation Time: 25 minutes Plus marinating time Cooking Time: 15 minutes

There is a lot of football watching in our house between my hot husband and my sports-crazed son. The lads settle in to watch their favourite teams (the Chargers, Patriots, and Packers), as well as the rest of the NFL. They don't want to chat much while the game is on, but I frequently hear "I'm hungry" and "Hey, are you going to make some snacks for the game?" " One of those football-watching Sundays when my boys were craving sweet chicken wings, I came up with this recipe. These are certainly sweet and sticky. They get a taste boost from the fresh cilantro sprinkled on top.

MARINADE

a third cup of soy sauce

14 cup dark brown sugar, packed

a quarter-cup of honey

1 tablespoon garlic, minced (about 3 large cloves)

1 tablespoon lemon juice, freshly squeezed

1 tablespoon fresh ginger, minced

1 teaspoon black pepper, freshly ground

THE FINAL INGREDIENTS

4 pound trimmed chicken wings (see Tips)

14 cup fresh cilantro, chopped

Combine all of the marinade ingredients in a big zip baggie. Seal the bag and stir the trimmed chicken wings and drumsticks around to coat them in the marinade. Refrigerate the marinating wings for at least 12 hours or overnight, flipping the bag occasionally to ensure that the marinade gets to all of the chicken pieces.

Preheat the oven to 450 degrees Fahrenheit. Place a baking rack on top of a rimmed baking sheet lined with foil. Using cooking spray, coat the rack.

The marinade should be drained and discarded from the bag. Arrange the chicken on the rack. Bake for 15 to 18 minutes, or until the skin of the chicken is dark brown and crispy. When the wings are pierced with a knife, the juices should run clear. Transfer the chicken to a serving plate and top with cilantro.

GLUTEN-FREE ADAPTABLE Use a gluten-free soy sauce brand.

TIP To trim chicken wings: Use a sharp knife or kitchen scissors to clip off and discard the tips. You'll wind up with a drumstick and a flat wing if you cut each wing at the joint.

This marinade is also wonderful when used on larger chicken drumsticks. Bake for 50 to 60 minutes at 350°F, or until chicken is cooked through.

Tots wrapped in bacon

Approximately 24 appetisers Time to Prepare: 25 minutes 15 minutes to prepare

The meal is perhaps the finest part of "Game Day," aside from watching those guys in tight trousers racing around the field with a football. It's usually about all kinds of comfort food, food for which you'd be prepared to sacrifice additional time at the gym, and food for which you only indulge once a year on Super Bowl Sunday. There are only four ingredients in this quick and easy appetiser recipe. It's fantastic for a football party, but it's also great for other times when you need some good ol' comfort food.

12 slices center-cut bacon, split crosswise in half

24 slightly defrosted tater tots (15 minutes at room temperature)

24 12-inch sharp cheddar cheese chunks

sauce Tabasco

toothpicks (24 total)

Preheat the oven to 450 degrees Fahrenheit. Use parchment paper or nonstick spray to line a baking pan.

On a level surface, place a piece of bacon. On top, place a tater tot. Cut a slit through the centre of the tater tot using a sharp knife. Insert a cheese slice through the slit. Sprinkle with Tabasco sauce. Wrap the bacon around the tater tots tightly and fasten with a toothpick. Rep with the rest of the ingredients.

Bake for 15 minutes, or until the tater tots are crispy and the bacon is cooked through. Serve right away.

ADAPTABLE WITHOUT GLUTEN Make sure to use gluten-free tater tots and bacon.

TIP Serve with a spicy sour cream dip made with sour cream and a pinch of Tabasco sauce.

MAKE-AHEAD SUGGESTIONS Place these on a baking sheet and assemble them a few hours ahead of time. Cover with plastic wrap and chill until ready to bake.

On top of the cheese, place a pickle slice.

To add a sweet flavour, roll the bacon-wrapped tater tots in brown sugar before baking; just be careful not to overbake them or the sugar will burn.

Cream cheese and a piece of peperoncini can be substituted for the cheddar cheese.

Chapter Twenty-nine

Mini corn dog muffins

This recipe makes 24 small muffins. Time to Prepare: 25 minutes 10 minutes to prepare

In our community, we host a lot of outdoor parties in a common area where the parents can mingle while the kids run wild. I always bring hundreds of these portable small muffins to contribute, and they fast disappear from the table. Dads and their kids frequently fight over who gets the last corn dog muffin.

cornmeal, 1 cup

12 cup flour (all-purpose)

2 tbsp. light brown sugar, packed

1 tablespoon powdered sugar

1 tblsp. salt

12 teaspoon bicarbonate of soda

1 gallon buttermilk

½ cup milk

2 teaspoons melted unsalted butter

1 egg, big

1 cup extra-sharp cheddar cheese, shredded

5 diced hot dogs

Optional dipping sauces: ketchup, mustard, sour cream, and/or honey mustard

Preheat the oven to 400 degrees Fahrenheit. Using shortening or nonstick spray, grease a 24-cup mini muffin pan thoroughly.

Whisk together the cornmeal, flour, sugar, baking powder, salt, and baking soda in a medium mixing basin.

Combine the buttermilk, milk, butter, and egg in a large mixing basin. Combine the dry ingredients and cheese in a small mixing bowl. Fill each muffin tray with a full tablespoon of batter. Fill each muffin cup with a couple pieces of hot dog.

10 to 12 minutes, or until golden brown Allow the muffins to cool in the pan for 10 to 15 minutes before removing them (see Tips). Warm with dipping sauces of choice.

TIP Slide a sharp knife between the outsides of the muffins and the pan, working the knife around the pan, then invert the pan upside down onto a big chopping board and yank the muffins out by tapping the bottoms of the muffin tins with the knife. They should easily slide out.

Chapter Thirty

In place of homemade cornmeal, use your favourite cornbread mix. Follow the package directions, adding 1 cup of cheddar cheese and chopped hot dogs as well. Add 2 tablespoons brown sugar to your favourite cornbread mix if it isn't sweet enough.

Chapter Thirty-one

Pull-apart bread with cheesy pepperoni pizza

1 huge bread loaf as an appetiser 20-minute prep time 30 minutes to prepare

In 2012, food blogs blossomed with recipes for pull-apart circular bread loaf. People split open their sourdough rounds and stuffed them with cheese, caramelised onions, mushrooms, and even ranch dressing, then baked them into a giant cheesy, wonderful mess of an appetiser, which became an Internet sensation. I, too, have jumped on the pull-apart bread bandwagon. It's the ideal appetiser to serve in front of a group of hungry individuals and let them help themselves. To hold it all together, I used diced pepperoni and pizza sauce, as well as a suitable amount of mozzarella and melted garlic butter.

1 loaf of French or sourdough bread, 20 oz.

1 cup pizza sauce from a jar

2 cups (8 ounces) mozzarella cheese, shredded

1 cup shredded cheddar cheese (4 ounces)

1 3.5-ounce box chopped sliced pepperoni (about 1 cup)

2 teaspoons melted salted butter

12 teaspoon powdered garlic

a quarter teaspoon of Italian seasoning

Optional extra pizza sauce, warmed for dipping

Preheat the oven to 350 degrees Fahrenheit.

On a cutting board, place the bread. Cut a crisscross pattern in the bread with a bread knife, leaving 12 inch between cuts and slicing down toward the bottom of the loaf without cutting through the bottom crust.

Place the bread loaf into a wide sheet of foil large enough to wrap around the loaf completely. Fill the cuts with pizza sauce. Combine the cheeses in a medium mixing basin. Also stuff the cuts with cheese and pepperoni. It'll be sloppy and imperfect, which is fine. Continue stuffing until all of the cheese and pepperoni has been used up, filling as many cuts as possible. In a small bowl, combine the butter, garlic powder, and Italian seasoning. Drizzle the sauce over the bread. Wrap the loaf in foil and bake it for 15 minutes. Remove the foil and bake for

15 to 20 minutes longer, or until the bread is toasted and the cheese has melted. Transfer the bread to a serving tray and serve immediately with a side of hot pizza sauce for dipping, if desired.

TIP It's fine to use a rectangular-shaped loaf if you can't find a round loaf. Simply buy one that isn't sliced and cross-cut it in the same manner.

Remove the pizza sauce and pepperoni and replace with 12 pound diced and cooked bacon. Drizzle with 4 tablespoons melted butter and 12 teaspoon garlic powder, then top with 12 cup green onions.

Chapter Thirty-two

toasted maple almonds with a kick

2 cup serving Time to Prepare: 25 minutes 15 minutes to prepare

If I were stranded on a desert island and the only food available was almonds, I believe I would be content. Almonds are my worst enemy. If it were okay, I'd eat them all day and in any way possible. All variations appeal to me, whether plain, naked, Marcona, roasted, spicy, or sweet. If you put a bowl of almonds in front of me, I'm not going to share them. But I'll share them with you. These almonds are roasted with sugared sweet maple syrup and melted butter, with a dash of cayenne pepper thrown in for good measure.

1 tablespoon white granulated sugar

1 teaspoon fine sea salt (distributed)

2 tablespoons butter, unsalted

2 tsp. maple syrup

2 cups almonds, blanched or raw

12 teaspoon chilli powder

Preheat the oven to 350 degrees Fahrenheit. Using nonstick spray, coat a 20-inch sheet of foil. Using nonstick spray, coat a baking sheet.

Combine the sugar and 12 teaspoon of salt in a small mixing dish. Place aside.

Heat the butter and syrup in a big skillet over medium-high heat until it's bubbling. Remove the pan from the heat and add the almonds and cayenne pepper. Toss to evenly coat. Place the almonds on the baking sheet that has been prepared. Spread the sugar mixture evenly over the nuts. Bake for 15 to 20 minutes, stirring halfway through, or until golden brown. Spread the almonds out as much as possible on the prepared foil. Allow it cool completely before storing in an airtight container.

ADAPTABLE WITHOUT GLUTEN Make sure to use a gluten-free maple syrup.

TIPS Walnuts, cashews, pecans, and other nuts work well in this dish.

You may make these almonds up to three days ahead of time. Keep them in an airtight container.

Don’t care for the heat? Instead of cayenne, use ground cinnamon.

Include herbs! 1 tablespoon coarsely chopped rosemary can be added to the skillet.

CPSIA information can be obtained
at www.ICGtesting.com
Printed in the USA
LVHW061835130722
723448LV00014B/174

9 781804 768365